AF255453

Air Fryer Toaster Oven Quick Recipes

Enjoy These Amazing Air Fryer Toaster Oven Recipes For Daily Healthy Meals

Eva Morris

TABLE OF CONTENT

this book has been derived from various sources. Please consult a licensed professional before attempting any techniques outlined in this book.

By reading this document, the reader agrees that under no circumstances is the author responsible for any losses, direct or indirect, which are incurred as a result of the use of information contained within this document, including, but not limited to, — errors, omissions, or inaccuracies.

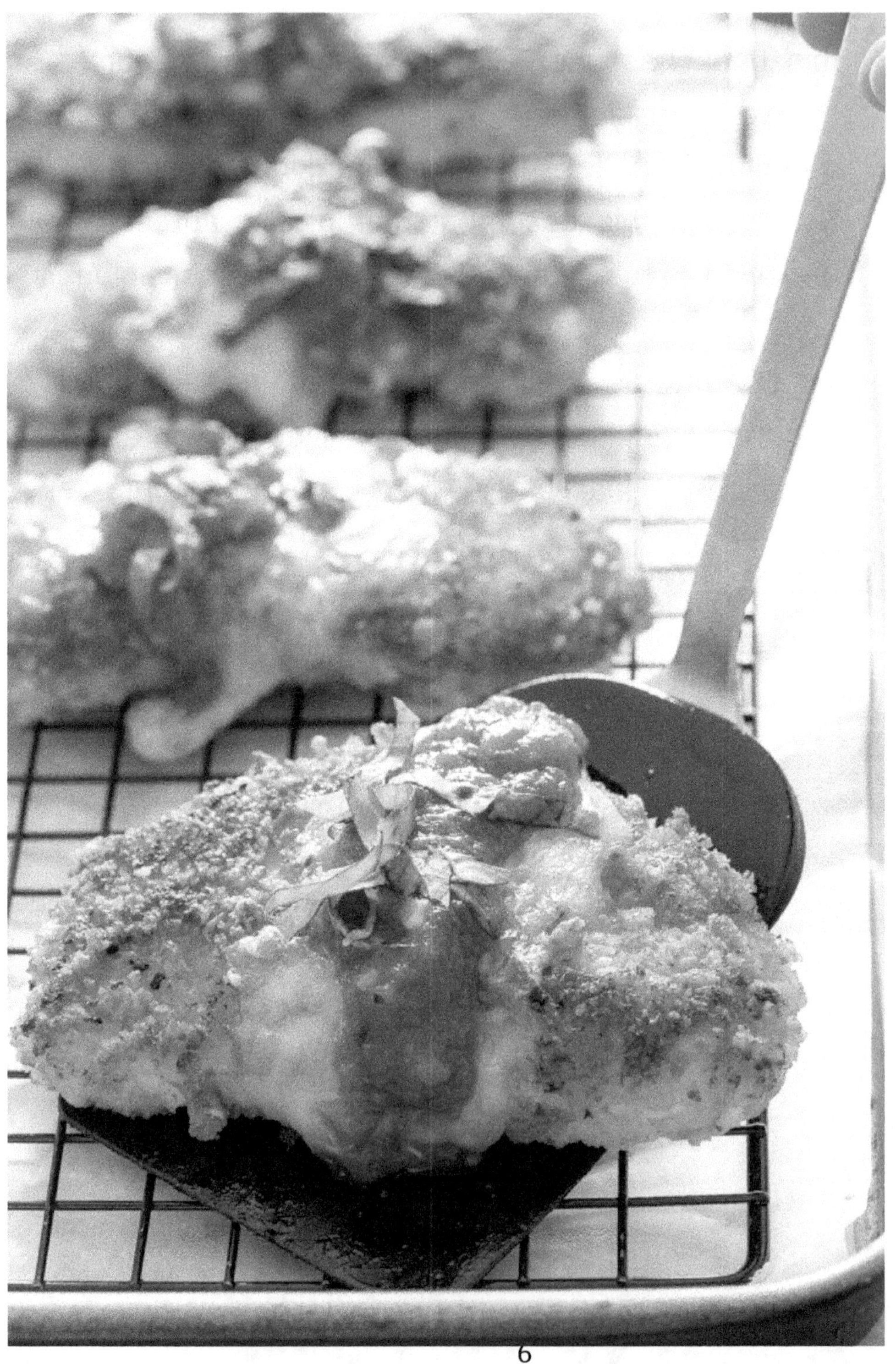

Perfect Chicken Parmesan

Preparation Time: 5minutes

Cooking Time: 225 minutes

Serving: 2

Ingredients

- Two sizeable white meat chicken breasts, approximately 5-6 ounces

- 1 cup of breadcrumbs (Panko brand works well)

- Two medium-sized eggs

- Pinch of salt and pepper

- One tablespoon of dried oregano

- 1 cup of marinara sauce (store-bought or homemade will do equally well)

- Two slices of provolone cheese

- One tablespoon of parmesan cheese

Directions:

1. Cover the air fryer's basket with a lining of tin foil, leaving the edges uncovered to

allow air to circulate through the basket.

2. Preheat the air fryer oven to 350 degrees.

3. In a mixing bowl, beat the eggs until fluffy until the yolks and whites are thoroughly combined, and set aside.

4. In a separate mixing bowl, combine the breadcrumbs, oregano, salt, and pepper, and set aside.

5. One by one, dip the raw chicken breasts into the bowl with dry ingredients, coating both sides, submerging into the bowl with wet ingredients, and then fall again into the dry ingredients. This double coating will ensure an extra crisp-and-delicious air-fry!

6. Lay the coated chicken breasts on the foil covering the air fryer basket in a single flat layer.

7. Set the air fryer timer for 10 minutes.

8. After 10 minutes, the air fryer will turn off, and the chicken should be mid-way cooked and the breaded coating starting to brown.

9. Using tongs, turn each piece of chicken over to ensure a full all-over fry.

10. Reset the air fryer to 320 degrees for another 10 minutes.

11. While the chicken is cooking, pour half the marinara sauce into a 7-inch heat-safe pan.

12. After 15 minutes, when the air fryer shuts off, remove the fried chicken breasts using tongs and set in the marinara-covered pan. Drizzle the rest of the marinara sauce over the fried chicken, then place the slices of provolone cheese atop both of them and sprinkle the parmesan cheese over the entire pan.

13. Reset the air fryer to 350 degrees for 5 minutes.

14. After 5 minutes, when the air fryer shuts off, remove the dish from the air fryer using tongs or oven mitts. The chicken will be perfectly crisped and the cheese melted and lightly toasted. Serve while hot!

Basil-Garlic Breaded Chicken Bake

Preparation Time: 5 minutes

Cooking Time: 30 minutes

Serving: 2

Ingredients

- Two boneless skinless chicken breast halves (4 ounces each)
- One tablespoon butter, melted
- One large tomato, seeded and chopped
- Two garlic cloves, minced
- 1 1/2 tablespoons minced fresh basil
- 1/2 tablespoon olive oil
- 1/2 teaspoon salt
- 1/4 cup all-purpose flour
- 1/4 cup egg substitute
- 1/4 cup grated Parmesan cheese

- 1/4 cup dry bread crumbs

- 1/4 teaspoon pepper

Directions:

1. In a shallow bowl, whisk OK egg substitute and place flour in a separate bowl—dip chicken in flour, then egg, and then flour. In a small bowl, whisk OK butter, bread crumbs, and cheese. Sprinkle over chicken.

2. Lightly grease the baking pan of the air fryer with cooking spray. Place breaded chicken on the bottom of the pan. Cover with foil.

3. For 20 minutes, cook at 390°F.

4. Meanwhile, in a bowl, whisk well-remaining ingredient.

5. Remove foil from pan and then pour over chicken the remaining Ingredients.

6. Cook for 8 minutes.

7. Serve and enjoy.

PER SERVING: CALORIES: 311; FAT: 11G; PROTEIN: 31G; CARBS: 22G

Buffalo Chicken Wings

Preparation Time: 5 minutes

Cooking Time: 30 minutes

Serving: 8

Ingredients

- 1 tsp. salt
- 1-2 tbsp. brown sugar
- 1 tbsp. Worcestershire sauce
- ½ C. vegan butter
- ½ C. cayenne pepper sauce
- 4 pounds of chicken wings

Directions:

1. Whisk salt, brown sugar, Worcestershire sauce, butter, and hot sauce together and set aside.

2. Dry wings and add to the air fryer basket.

3. Set temperature to 380°F, and set time to 25 minutes. Cook was tossing halfway through.

4. When the timer sounds, shake wings, bump up the temperature to 400 degrees, and cook another 5 minutes.

5. Take out wings and place them into a big bowl. Add sauce and toss well.

6. Serve alongside celery sticks.

Nutrition: CALORIES: 402; FAT: 16G; PROTEIN: 17G; SUGAR: 4G

Zingy & Nutty Chicken Wings

Preparation Time: 5 minutes

Cooking Time: 18 minutes

Serving: 4

Ingredients

- One tablespoon fish sauce

- One tablespoon fresh lemon juice

- One teaspoon sugar

- 12 chicken middle wings, cut into half

- Two fresh lemongrass stalks, chopped finely

- ¼ cup unsalted cashews, crushed

Directions:

1. In a bowl, mix fish sauce, lime juice, and sugar.

2. Add wings ad coat with mixture generously. Refrigerate to marinate for

about 1-2 hours.

3. Preheat the air fryer oven to 355 degrees F.

4. In the air fryer oven pan, place lemongrass stalks—Cook for about 2-3 minutes. Remove the cashew mixture from Air fryer and transfer it into a bowl. Now, set the air fryer oven to 390 degrees F.

5. Place the chicken wings in the air fryer pan. Cook for about 13-15 minutes further.

6. Transfer the wings into serving plates. Sprinkle with cashew mixture and serve.

Honey And Wine Chicken Breasts

Preparation Time: 15 minutes

Cooking Time: 20 minutes

Serving: 4

Ingredients

- Two chicken breasts, rinsed and halved

- One tablespoon melted butter

- 1/2 teaspoon freshly ground pepper, or to taste

- 3/4 teaspoon sea salt, or to taste

- One teaspoon paprika

- One teaspoon dried rosemary

- Two tablespoons dry white wine

- One tablespoon honey

Directions:

1. Firstly, pat the chicken breasts dry. Lightly coat them with the melted butter.

2. Then, add the remaining ingredients.

3. Transfer them to the air fryer basket; bake about 15 minutes at 330 degrees F. Serve warm and enjoy!

Nutrition:

CALORIES: 189;

FAT: 14G;

PROTEIN: 11G;

SUGAR: 1G

Chicken Fillets, Brie & Ham

Preparation Time: 5 minutes

Cooking Time: 15 minutes

Serving: 4

Ingredients

- 2 Large Chicken Fillets
- Freshly Ground Black Pepper
- 4 Small Slices of Brie (Or your cheese of choice)
- 1 Tbsp. Freshly Chopped Chives
- 4 Slices Cured Ham

Directions:

1. Slice the fillets into four and make incisions as you would for a hamburger bun. Leave a little "hinge" uncut at the back. Season the inside and pop some brie and chives in there. Close them, and wrap them each in a slice of ham. Brush with oil and pop them into the basket.

2. Heat your fryer to 350° F. Pour into the Oven rack/basket. Place the Rack on the middle-shelf of the Air fryer oven. Set temperature to 400°F, and set time to 15 minutes. Roast the little parcels until they look tasty (15 min)

Chicken Fajitas

Preparation Time: 10 minutes

Cooking Time: 20 minutes

Serving: 4

Ingredients

- Four boneless, skinless chicken breasts, sliced

- One small red onion, sliced

- Two red bell peppers, sliced

- ½ cup spicy ranch salad dressing, divided

- ½ teaspoon dried oregano

- Eight corn tortillas

- 2 cups torn butter lettuce

- • Two avocados, peeled and chopped

Directions:

1. Place the chicken, onion, and pepper in the air fryer basket. Drizzle with one tablespoon of the salad dressing and add the oregano. Toss to combine.

2. Place the Rack on the middle-shelf of the Air fryer oven. Set temperature to 165°F, and set time to 14 minutes. Grill for 10 to 14 minutes or until the chicken is 165°F on a food thermometer. Transfer the chicken and vegetables to a bowl and toss with the remaining salad dressing. Serve the chicken mixture with the tortillas, lettuce, and avocados and let everyone make their creations.

Nutrition: CALORIES: 783; FAT: 38G; PROTEIN: 72; FIBER: 12G

Crispy Honey Garlic Chicken Wings

Preparation Time: 10 minutes

Cooking Time: 25 minutes

Serving: 8

Ingredients

- 1/8 C. water
- ½ tsp. salt
- 4 tbsp. minced garlic
- ¼ C. vegan butter
- ¼ C. raw honey
- ¾ C. almond flour
- 16 chicken wings

Directions:

1. Rinse off and dry chicken wings well.

2. Spray air fryer basket with olive oil.

3. Coat chicken wings with almond flour and add coated attachments to the air fryer.

4. Pour into the Oven basket. Place the basket on the middle shelf of the Air fryer oven. Set temperature to 380°F, and set time to 25 minutes. Cook was shaking every 5 minutes.

5. When the timer goes off, cook 5-10 minutes at 400 degrees till the skin becomes crispy and dry.

6. As chicken cooks, melt butter in a saucepan and add garlic. Sauté garlic 5 minutes. Add salt and honey, simmer 20 minutes. Make sure to stir every so often so the sauce does not burn. Add a bit of water after 15 minutes to ensure the sauce does not harden.

7. Take out chicken wings from the air fryer and coat in sauce. Enjoy!

Nutrition: CALORIES: 435; FAT: 19G; PROTEIN: 31G; SUGAR: 6G

Chicken Stir-Fry

Preparation Time: 10 minutes

Cooking Time: 20 minutes

Servings: 2

Ingredients:

- 1 (6-oz. chicken breast; cut into 1-inch cubes
- ½ medium red bell pepper; seeded and chopped
- ½ medium zucchini; chopped
- ¼ medium red onion; peeled and sliced
- 1 tbsp. Coconut oil
- ½ tsp. Garlic powder.
- 1 tsp. Dried oregano.
- ¼ tsp. dried thyme

Directions:

1. Place all ingredients into a large mixing bowl and toss until the coconut oil coats the meat and vegetables. Pour the contents of the bowl into the air fryer

basket

2. Adjust the temperature to 375°F and set the timer for 15 minutes. Shake the fryer basket halfway through the cooking time to redistribute the food. Serve readily.

Nutrition:

Calories: 186 kcal/Cal

Protein: 20.4 g

Fiber: 1.7 g

Fat: 8.0 g

Carbohydrates: 5.6 g

Chicken Pizza Crust

Preparation Time: 10 minutes

Cooking Time: 25 minutes

Servings: 4

Ingredients:

- 1 lb. ground chicken thigh meat
- ½ cup shredded mozzarella
- ¼ cup grated Parmesan cheese.

Directions:

1. Take a large bowl, mix all ingredients. Separate into four even parts.

2. Cut out four (6-inch circles of parchment and press each part of the chicken mixture out onto one of the processes. Place into the air fryer basket, working in batches as needed

3. Adjust the temperature to 375°F and set the timer for 25 minutes. Flip the crust halfway through the cooking time

4. Once fully cooked, you may top it with cheese and your favorite toppings and cook five additional minutes. Or you may place crust into refrigerator or freezer and top when ready to eat.

Nutrition:

Calories: 230 kcal/Cal

Protein: 24.7 g

Fiber: 0.0 g

Fat: 12.8 g

Carbohydrates: 1.2 g

Spiced Chicken Breasts

Preparation Time: 15 minutes

Cooking Time: 10 minutes

Servings: 4

Ingredients:

- Four chicken breasts, skinless and boneless
- 1 tbsp. parsley; chopped
- 1 tsp. smoked paprika
- 1 tsp. garlic powder
- 1 tsp. chili powder
- A drizzle of olive oil
- A pinch of salt and black pepper

Directions:

1. Season chicken with salt and pepper and rub it with the oil and all the other ingredients except the parsley

2. Put the chicken breasts in your air fryer's basket and cook at 350°F for 10 minutes

on each side

3. Divide between plates, sprinkle the parsley
   on top, and serve

Nutrition:

Calories: 222 kcal/Cal

Fat: 11 g

Fiber: 4 g

Carbohydrates: 6 g

Protein: 12 g

Spiced Duck Legs

Preparation Time: 5 minutes

Cooking Time: 25 minutes

Servings: 4

Ingredients

- Two garlic cloves; minced

- 2 tbsp. olive oil

- 1 tsp. five-spice

- 1 tsp. hot chili powder

- A pinch of salt and black pepper

Directions:

1. Take a bowl and mix the duck legs with all the other ingredients and rub them well.

2. Put the duck legs in your air fryer's basket and cook at 380°F for 25 minutes, flipping them halfway

3. Divide between plates and serve!

Nutrition:

Calories: 287 kcal/Cal

Fat: 12g

Fiber: 4 g

Carbohydrates: 6 g

Protein: 17 g

Nutmeg Chicken Thighs

Preparation Time: 15 minutes

Cooking Time: 20 minutes

Servings: 4

Ingredients:

- 2 lb. chicken thighs
- 2 tbsp. Olive oil
- ½ tsp. nutmeg, ground
- A pinch of salt and black pepper

Directions:

1. Season the chicken thighs with salt and pepper and rub with the rest of the ingredients

2. Put the chicken thighs in the air fryer's basket, cook at 360°F for 15 minutes on each side, divide between plates and serve.

Nutrition:

Calories: 271 kcal/Cal

Fat: 12 g

Fiber: 4 g

Carbohydrates: 6 g

Protein: 13 g

Creamy Chicken Wings

Preparation Time: 5 minutes

Cooking Time: 30 minutes

Servings: 4

Ingredients:

- 2 lb. chicken wings
- ¼ cup parmesan, grated
- ½ cup heavy cream
- Three garlic cloves; minced
- 3 tbsp. Butter; melted
- ½ tsp. Oregano; dried
- ½ tsp. basil; dried
- Salt and black pepper to taste.

Directions:

1. In a baking dish that fits your air fryer, mix the chicken wings with all the ingredients except the parmesan and toss

2. Put the dish in your air fryer and cook at 380°F for 30 minutes. Sprinkle the cheese

on top, leave the mix aside for 10 minutes, divide between plates and serve

Nutrition:

Calories: 270 kcal/Cal

Fat: 12 g

Fiber: 3 g

Carbohydrates: 6 g

Protein: 17 g

Cheddar Turkey Bites

Preparation Time: 5 minutes

Cooking Time: 20 minutes

Servings: 4

Ingredients:

- One big turkey breast, skinless; boneless, and cubed
- 1 tbsp. Olive oil
- ¼ cup cheddar cheese, grated
- ¼ tsp. garlic powder
- Salt and black pepper to taste.

Directions:

1. Rub the turkey cubes with the oil, season with salt, pepper, garlic powder, and dredge in cheddar cheese.

2. Put the turkey bits in your air fryer's basket and cook at 380°F for 20 minutes. Divide between plates and serve with a side salad

Nutrition:

Calories: 240 kcal/Cal

Fat: 11 g

Fiber: 2 g

Carbohydrates: 5 g

Protein: 12 g

Chicken Parmesan

Preparation Time: 5 minutes

Cooking Time: 25 minutes

Servings: 4

Ingredients:

- 2 (6-oz. boneless, skinless chicken breasts

- 1 oz. Pork rinds, crushed

- ½ cup grated Parmesan cheese, divided.

- One cup low-carb, no-sugar-added pasta sauce

- One cup shredded mozzarella cheese, divided.

- 4 tbsp. Full-fat mayonnaise, divided.

- ½ tsp. Garlic powder.

- ¼ tsp. Dried oregano.

- ½ tsp. Dried parsley.

Directions:

1. Slice each chicken breast in half lengthwise and lb. out to 3/4-inch thickness. Sprinkle with garlic powder, oregano, and parsley.

2. Spread 1 tbsp. Mayonnaise on top of each piece of chicken and then sprinkle ¼ cup mozzarella on each piece.

3. In a small bowl, mix the crushed pork rinds and Parmesan. Sprinkle the mixture on top of mozzarella.

4. Pour sauce into a 6-inch round baking pan and place chicken on top. Place pan into the air fryer basket. Adjust the temperature to 320°F and set the timer for 25 minutes.

5. The cheese will be browned, and the internal temperature will be at least 165°F when fully cooked.

6. Serve warm.

Nutrition:

Calories: 393 kcal/Cal

Protein: 34.2 g

Fiber: 2.1 g

Fat: 22.8 g

Carbohydrates: 6.8 g

Lemon Pepper Drumsticks

Preparation Time: 5 minutes

Cooking Time: 25 minutes

Servings: 8 drumsticks

Ingredients:

- Eight chicken drumsticks

- 1 tbsp. lemon-pepper seasoning

- 4 tbsp. Salted butter; melted.

- 2 tsp. Baking powder.

- ½ tsp. Garlic powder.

Directions:

1. Sprinkle baking powder and garlic powder over drumsticks and rub into chicken skin —place drumsticks into the air fryer basket.

2. Adjust the temperature to 375°F and set the timer for 25 minutes

3. Use tongs to turn drumsticks halfway through the cooking time. When the skin is

golden, and the internal temperature is at least 165°F, remove from the fryer.

4. Take a large bowl, mix butter, and lemon pepper seasoning. Add drumsticks to the bowl and toss until coated.

5. Serve warm.

Nutrition:

Calories: 532 kcal/Cal

Protein: 48.3 g

Fiber: 0.0 g

Fat: 32.3

Carbohydrates: 1.2 g

Mustard Turkey Bites

Preparation Time: 5 minutes

Cooking Time: 20 minutes

Servings: 4

Ingredients:

- One big turkey breast, skinless; boneless, and cubed
- Four garlic cloves; minced
- 1 tbsp. mustard
- 1 ½ tbsp. olive oil
- Salt and black pepper to taste.

Directions:

1. Take a bowl and mix the chicken with the garlic and the other ingredients and toss.

2. Put the turkey in your air fryer's basket, cook at 360°F for 20 minutes, divide between plates and serve with a side salad

Nutrition:

Calories: 240 kcal/Cal

Fat: 12 g

Fiber: 4 g

Carbohydrates: 6 g

Protein: 15g

Turkey Turnovers

Preparation Time: 10 minutes

Cooking time: 10 minutes

Servings: 8

Ingredients:

- 2 cups turkey, cooked & chopped
- 1 cup cheddar cheese, grated
- 1 cup broccoli, cooked & chopped
- ½ cup mayonnaise
- ½ tsp. salt
- ¼ tsp. pepper
- Two cans of refrigerated crescent rolls

Directions:

1. Place the baking pan in position 1 of the oven.

2. In a large bowl, combine all ingredients, except rolls, mix well.

3. Separate each can of rolls into four squares, press perforations to seal.

4. Spoon turkey mixture in the center of each square. Fold over diagonally and seal the edges.

5. Set oven to bake at 375°F for 15 minutes.

6. Brush tops of turnovers lightly with additional mayonnaise. After the oven has preheated for 5 minutes, place turnovers on baking pan and cook 10-12 minutes or until golden brown; serve warm.

Nutrition:

Calories: 309 kcal/Cal

Total Fat: 21 g

Saturated Fat: 6 g

Cholesterol: 0 mg

Sodium: 0 mg

Total Carbs: 15 g

Fiber: 2 g

Sugar: 1 g

Protein: 15 g

Chicken Pram

Preparation Time: 10 minutes

Cooking time: 35 minutes

Servings: 4

Ingredients:

- Nonstick cooking spray
- ½ cup flour
- Two eggs
- 2/3 cup panko breadcrumbs
- 2/3 cup Italian seasoned breadcrumbs
- 1/3 + ¼ cup parmesan cheese, divided
- 2 tbsp. fresh parsley, chopped
- ½ tsp. salt
- ¼ tsp. pepper
- Four chicken breast halves, skinless & boneless
- 24 oz. marinara sauce

- 1 cup mozzarella cheese, grated

Directions:

1. Place the baking pan in position 2 of the oven. Lightly spray the fryer basket with cooking spray.

2. Place flour in a shallow dish.

3. In a separate shallow dish, beat the eggs.

4. In a third shallow dish, combine both breadcrumbs, 1/3 cup parmesan cheese, two tablespoons parsley, salt, and pepper.

5. Place chicken between two sheets of plastic wrap and pound to ½-inch thick.

6. Dip chicken first in flour, then eggs, and breadcrumb mixture to coat. Place in the basket and then put the basket on the baking pan.

7. Set oven to air fry on 375°F for 10 minutes. Turn chicken over halfway through cooking time.

8. Remove chicken and baking pan from the oven. Place the rack in position 1. Set range to bake on 425°F for 30 minutes.

9. Pour 1 ½ cups marinara in the bottom of an 8x11-inch baking dish. Place chicken over the sauce and add another two tablespoons marinara to tops of chicken. Top the chicken with mozzarella and parmesan cheese once oven preheats for 5 minutes, place the dish in the oven and bake 20-25 minutes until bubbly and cheese is golden brown. Serve.

Nutrition:

Calories: 529 kcal/Cal

Total Fat: 13 g

Saturated Fat: 5 g

Cholesterol: 0 mg

Sodium: 1437 mg

Total Carbs: 52 g

Fiber: 5 g

Sugar: 9 g

Protein: 51 g

Teriyaki Duck Legs

Preparation Time: 15 minutes

Cooking time: 2 hours

Servings: 6

Ingredients:

- 3 lbs. duck legs
- ½ cup teriyaki sauce
- 2 tbsp. soy sauce
- 2 tbsp. malt vinegar

Directions:

1. Place the rack in position 1 of the oven.

2. Place the duck legs, skin side up, in an 8x11-inch baking dish.

3. In a small bowl, whisk together the remaining ingredients and pour around duck legs. The liquid needs to reach the skin level. If not, add water until it does.

4. Set the oven to convection bake at 300°F for 60 minutes. After 5 minutes, place the

ducks in the range and cook 90 minutes, or until tender.

5. Remove duck from the oven. Pour off cooking liquid into a small saucepan. Skim off fat and reserve. Bring sauce to a boil and cook until it reduces, about 10 minutes, stirring occasionally.

6. Place the baking pan in position 2 of the oven. Place the duck legs in the fryer basket and brush with reserved fat and sauce. Place the basket in the oven and set to broil at 400°F for 10 minutes. Turn duck over halfway through and brush with fat and sauce again. Serve.

Nutrition:

Calories: 608 kcal/Cal

Total Fat: 20 g

Saturated Fat: 5 g

Cholesterol: 0 mg

Sodium: 1063 mg

Total Carbs: 6 g

Fiber: 0 g

Sugar: 5 g

Protein: 101 g

Crunchy Almond & Kale Salad With Roasted Chicken

Preparation Time: 10 minutes

Cooking Time: 20 minutes

Servings: 1

Ingredients:

- Salad

- 1 teaspoon extra virgin olive oil

- 100g Lacinato kale, sliced into thin strips

- 1/4 cup roasted almonds

- Pinch of sea salt

- Pinch of pepper

- Roasted Chicken

- 100g chicken thighs

- Pinch of sea salt

- Pinch of pepper

- 1 teaspoon apple cider vinegar

- 1/2 teaspoon extra-virgin olive oil

- 1 tablespoon rosemary

- 1 tablespoon cup sage

Directions:

1. Place kale in a bowl and add olive oil; massage olive oil with hands into the kale until kale is tender; sprinkle with salt and pepper and toss with toasted almonds.

2. Preheat your air fryer toast oven to 360°F.

3. Sprinkle chicken with salt and pepper; add vinegar and olive oil and season with rosemary and sage.

4. Roast in the basket of your air fryer toast oven for about 20 minutes, turning the chicken halfway through or until chicken is cooked through.

5. Serve chicken with kale and almond salad.

Nutrition:

Calories: 293 kcal,

Carbs: 10 g,

Fat: 16.4 g,

Golden Beer-Battered Cod

Preparation Time: 5minutes

Cooking time: 15 minutes

Servings: 4

Ingredients:

- Two eggs
- 1 cup malty beer
- 1 cup all-purpose flour
- ½ cup cornstarch
- One teaspoon garlic powder
- Salt and pepper, to taste
- 4 (4-ounce / 113-g) cod fillets
- Cooking spray

Directions:

1. In a shallow bowl, beat together the eggs with the beer. In another shallow bowl, thoroughly combine the flour and cornstarch. Sprinkle with the garlic powder, salt, and pepper.

2. Dredge each cod fillet in the flour mixture, then in the egg mixture. Dip each piece of fish in the flour mixture a second time.

3. Spritz the air fry basket with cooking spray. Arrange the cod fillets in the basket in a single layer.

4. Select Air Fry, Convection, set temperature to 400ºF (205ºC), and set time to 15 minutes. Select Start to begin preheating.

5. Once preheated, place the basket on the air fry position. Flip the fillets halfway through the cooking time.

6. When cooking is complete, the cod should reach an internal temperature of 145ºF (63ºC) on a meat thermometer, and the outside should be crispy. Let the fish cool for 5 minutes and serve.

Sticky Hoisin Tuna

Preparation Time: 15minutes

Cooking time: 5 minutes

Servings: 4

Ingredients:

- ½ cup hoisin sauce

- 2tablespoons rice wine vinegar

- 2 teaspoons sesame oil

- 2 teaspoons dried lemongrass

- 1teaspoon garlic powder

- ¼ teaspoon red pepper flakes

- ½ small onion, quartered and thinly sliced

- ounces (227 g) fresh tuna, cut into 1-inch cubes

- •   Cooking spray

- •   3cups cooked jasmine rice

Directions:

1. In a small bowl, whisk together the hoisin sauce, vinegar, sesame oil, lemongrass, garlic powder, and red pepper flakes.

2. Add the sliced onion and tuna cubes and gently toss until the fish is evenly coated.

3. Arrange the coated tuna cubes in the air fry basket in a single layer.

4. Select Air Fry, Convection, set temperature to 390ºF (199ºC), and set time to 5 minutes. Select Start to begin preheating.

5. Once preheated, place the basket on the air fry position. Flip the fish halfway through the cooking time.

6. When cooking is complete, the fish should begin to flake. Continue cooking for 1 minute, if necessary. Remove from the oven and serve over hot jasmine rice.

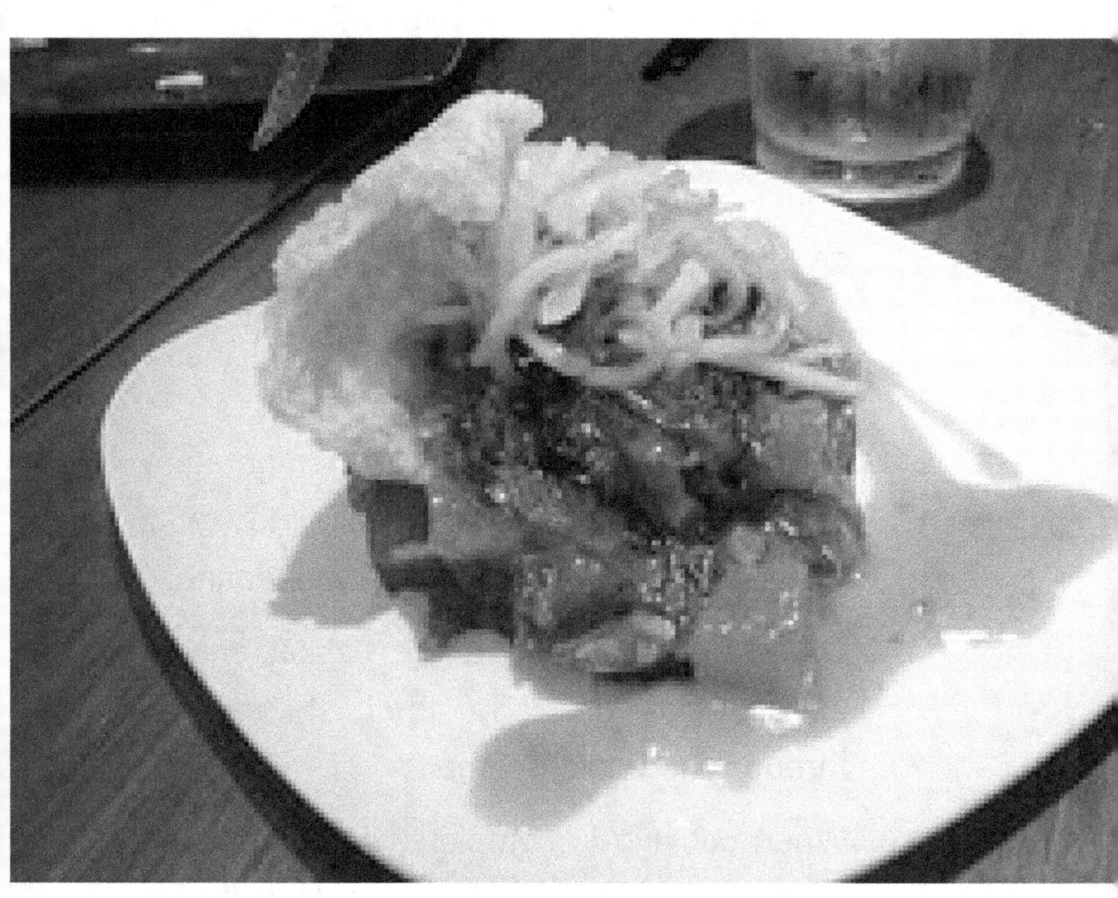

Parmesan-Crusted Halibut Fillets

Preparation Time: 5minutes

Cooking time: 10 minutes

Servings: 4

Ingredients:

- 2medium-sized halibut fillets

- Dash of Tabasco sauce

- 1teaspoon curry powder

- ½ teaspoon ground coriander

- ½ teaspoon hot paprika

- Kosher salt and freshly cracked mixed peppercorns, to taste

- **2eggs**

- 1½ tablespoons olive oil

- ½ cup grated Parmesan cheese

Directions:

1. On a clean work surface, drizzle the halibut fillets with the Tabasco sauce. Sprinkle with the curry powder, coriander, hot

paprika, salt, and cracked mixed peppercorns. Set aside.

2. In a shallow bowl, beat the eggs until frothy. In another shallow bowl, combine the olive oil and Parmesan cheese.

3. One at a time, dredge the halibut fillets in the beaten eggs, shaking off any excess, then roll them over the Parmesan cheese until evenly coated.

4. Arrange the halibut fillets in the air fry basket in a single layer.

5. Select Roast, Convection, set temperature to 365ºF (185ºC), and set time to 10 minutes. Select Start to begin preheating.

6. Once preheated, place the basket on the roast position.

7. When cooking is complete, the fish should be golden brown and crisp. Cool for 5 minutes before serving.

Tilapia Meniere With Vegetables

Preparation time: 10 minutes

Cooking time: 20 minutes

Servings: 4

Ingredients:

- 10 ounces (283 g) Yukon Gold potatoes, sliced ¼-inch thick

- Five tablespoons unsalted butter, melted, divided

- One teaspoon kosher salt, divided

- 4 (8-ounce / 227-g) tilapia fillets

- ½ pound (227 g) green beans, trimmed

- Juice of 1 lemon

- Two tablespoons chopped fresh parsley, for garnish

Directions:

1. Drizzle the potatoes with two tablespoons of melted butter and ¼ teaspoon of kosher

salt in a large bowl. Transfer the potatoes to the sheet pan.

2. Select Roast, Convection, set temperature to 375ºF (190ºC), and set time to 20 minutes.

3. Meanwhile, season both sides of the fillets with ½ teaspoon of kosher salt. Put the green beans in the medium bowl and sprinkle with the remaining ¼ teaspoon of kosher salt and one tablespoon of butter, tossing to coat.

4. After 10 minutes, remove the pan and push the potatoes to one side. Put the fillets in the middle of the pan and add the green beans on the other side.

5. Drizzle the rest of the two tablespoons of butter over the fillets. Return it and cook until the fish flakes easily with a fork, and the green beans are crisp-tender.

6. Once cooked, remove and drizzle the lemon juice over the fillets and sprinkle the parsley on top for garnish. Serve hot.

Nutrition:

Calories: 172

Carbs: 24g

Fat: 2g

Protein: 24g

Glazed Tuna And Fruit Kebabs

Preparation time: 15 minutes

Cooking time: 10 minutes

Servings: 4

Ingredients:

Kebabs:

- 1-pound (454 g) tuna steaks, cut into 1-inch cubes

- ½ cup canned pineapple chunks, drained, juice reserved

- ½ cup large red grapes

Marinade:

- One tablespoon honey

- One teaspoon olive oil

- Two teaspoons grated fresh ginger

- Pinch cayenne pepper

- Special Equipment:

- Four metal skewers

Directions:

1. Make the kebabs: Thread, alternating tuna cubes, pineapple chunks, and red grapes, onto the metal skewers.

2. Make the marinade: Whisk the honey, olive oil, ginger, and cayenne pepper in a small bowl. Brush the marinade generously over the kebabs and allow them to sit for 10 minutes.

3. When ready, transfer the kebabs to the air fry basket.

4. Select Air Fry, Convection, set temperature to 370ºF (188ºC), and set time to 10 minutes.

5. After 5 minutes, remove and flip the kebabs and brush with the remaining marinade. Return the basket to the oven and continue cooking for an additional 5 minutes.

6. Remove, and discard any remaining marinade. Serve hot.

Nutrition:

Calories: 319

Carbs: 0g

Fat: 0g

Protein: 0g

Snapper With Tomatoes And Olives

Preparation time: 9 minutes

Cooking time: 18 minutes

Servings: 4

Ingredients:

- Two tablespoons extra-virgin olive oil

- Two large garlic cloves, minced

- ½ onion, finely chopped

- 1 (14.5-ounce / 411-g) can diced tomatoes, drained

- ¼ cup sliced green olives

- Three tablespoons capers, divided

- Two tablespoons chopped fresh parsley, divided

- ½ teaspoon dried oregano

- 4 (6-ounce / 170-g) snapper fillets

- ½ teaspoon kosher salt

Directions:

1. Grease the sheet pan generously with olive oil, and then place the pan on the roast position.

2. Select Roast, Convection, set temperature to 375ºF (190ºC), and set time to 18 minutes.

3. Remove the pan and add the garlic and onion to the pan's olive oil, stirring to coat, then return it to the air fryer oven. Set within 2 minutes.

4. Remove, and then stir in the tomatoes, olives, 1½ tablespoons of capers, one tablespoon of parsley, and oregano. Return it and cook within 6 minutes until heated through.

5. Meanwhile, rub the fillets with the salt on both sides.

6. After another 6 minutes, remove and put the fillets in the center of the sheet pan, and spoon it. Return it and continue cooking, or until the fish is flaky.

7. When cooked, remove and scatter the remaining 1½ tablespoons of capers and one tablespoon of parsley on top of the fillets, then serve.

Nutrition:

Calories: 328

Carbs: 4g

Fat: 16g

Protein: 36g

Air Fried Cod Fillets

Preparation time: 15 minutes

Cooking time: 12 minutes

Servings: 4

Ingredients:

- Four cod fillets
- ¼ teaspoon acceptable sea salt
- One teaspoon cayenne pepper
- ¼ teaspoon ground black pepper
- ½ cup fresh Italian parsley, coarsely chopped
- ½ cup non-dairy milk
- Four garlic cloves, minced
- 1 Italian pepper, chopped
- One teaspoon dried basil
- ½ teaspoon dried oregano
- Cooking spray

Directions:

1. Lightly grease a baking dish using cooking spray.

2. Season the fillets with salt, cayenne pepper, and black pepper.

3. Pulse the remaining ingredients in a food processor and then transfer the mixture to a shallow bowl. Coat the fillets with the mixture.

4. Select Air Fry, Convection, set temperature to 375ºF (190ºC), and set time to 12 minutes.

5. Remove once it's done and serve on a plate.

Nutrition:

Calories: 80

Carbs: 0g

Fat: 3g

Protein: 14g

Crispy Fish Sticks

Preparation time: 10 minutes

Cooking time: 6 minutes

Servings: 8

Ingredients:

- 8 ounces (227 g) fish fillets (Pollock or cod), cut into ½ × 3 inches strips
- Salt, to taste (optional)
- ½ cup plain bread crumbs
- Cooking spray

Directions:

1. Season the fish strips with salt to taste, if desired.

2. Put the bread crumbs on a plate, and then roll the fish in the bread crumbs until well coated. Spray all sides of the fish with cooking spray. Transfer to the air fry basket in a single layer.

3. Select Air Fry, Convection, set temperature to 400ºF (205ºC), and set time to 6 minutes.

4. When cooked, the fish sticks should be golden brown and crispy. Serve hot.

Nutrition:

Calories: 220

Carbs: 20g

Fat: 10g

Protein: 11g

Fried Calamari

Preparation Time: 8minutes

Cooking Time: 7 minutes

Serving: 7

Ingredients

- ½ tsp. salt

- ½ tsp. Old Bay seasoning

- 1/3 C. plain cornmeal

- ½ C. semolina flour

- ½ C. almond flour

- 5-6 C. olive oil

- 1½ pounds baby squid

Directions:

1. Rinse squid in cold water and slice tentacles, keeping just ¼-inch of the hood in one piece.

2. Combine 1-2 pinches of pepper, salt, Old Bay seasoning, cornmeal, and both flours. Dredge squid pieces into the flour mixture and place it into the air fryer basket.

3. Spray liberally with olive oil. Cook 15 minutes at 345 degrees till coating turns a golden brown.

Nutrition:

CALORIES: 211; CARBS: 55; FAT: 6G; PROTEIN: 21G; SUGAR: 1G

Soy And Ginger Shrimp

Preparation Time: 8 minutes

Cooking Time: 10 minutes

Serving: 4

Ingredients

- Two tablespoons olive oil
- 2tablespoons scallions, finely chopped
- 2cloves garlic, chopped
- teaspoon fresh ginger, grated
- One tablespoon dry white wine
- One tablespoon balsamic vinegar
- 1/4 cup soy sauce
- tablespoon sugar
- 1 pound shrimp
- Salt and ground black pepper, to taste

Directions:

1. To make the marinade, warm the oil in a saucepan; cook all ingredients, except the shrimp, salt, and black pepper. Now, let it cool.

2. Marinate the shrimp, covered, at least an hour, in the refrigerator.

3. After that, pour into the Oven rack/basket. Place the Rack on the middle-shelf of the Smart Air Fryer Oven. Set temperature to 350°F, and set time to 10 minutes. Bake the shrimp at 350 degrees F for 8 to 10 minutes (depending on the size), turning once or twice. Season prepared shrimp with salt and black pepper and serve.

Crispy Cheesy Fish Fingers

Preparation Time: 10 minutes

Cooking Time: 20 minutes

Serving: 4

Ingredients

- Large codfish filet, approximately 6-8 ounces, fresh or frozen and thawed, cut into one ½-inch strip

- 2raw eggs

- ½ cup of breadcrumbs (we like Panko, but any brand or home recipe will do)

- 2tablespoons of shredded or powdered parmesan cheese

- 1tablespoons of shredded cheddar cheese

- Pinch of salt and pepper

Directions:

1. Cover the Smart Air Fryer Oven basket with a lining of tin foil, leaving the edges uncovered to allow air to circulate through the basket.

1. Preheat the Smart Air Fryer Oven to 350 degrees.

2. In a large mixing bowl, beat the eggs until fluffy until the yolks and whites are thoroughly combined.

3. Dunk all the fish strips in the beaten eggs, fully submerging.

4. In a separate mixing bowl, combine the bread crumbs with the parmesan, cheddar, salt, and pepper until evenly mixed.

5. One by one, coat the egg-covered fish strips in the mixed dry ingredients so that they're fully covered, and place on the foil-lined air fryer basket.

2. Set the Smart Air Fryer Oven timer to 20 minutes.

6. Halfway through the cooking time, shake the air fryer's handle so that the breaded fish jostles inside and fry coverage is even.

7. After 20 minutes, when the fryer shuts off, the fish strips will be perfectly cooked, and

their breaded crust golden-brown and delicious! Using tongs, remove from the air fryer and set on a serving dish to cool.

Panko-Crusted Tilapia

Preparation Time: 5 minutes

Cooking Time: 10 minutes

Serving: 3

Ingredients

- 2tsp. Italian seasoning

- 2 tsp. lemon pepper

- 1/3 C. panko breadcrumbs

- 1/3 C. egg whites

- 1/3 C. almond flour

- 3tilapia fillets

- Olive oil

Directions:

1. Place panko, egg whites, and flour into separate bowls: mix lemon pepper and Italian seasoning with breadcrumbs.

2. Pat tilapia fillets dry. Dredge in flour, then egg, breadcrumb mixture.

3. Add to the air fryer basket and spray lightly with olive oil.

4. Cook 10-11 minutes at 400 degrees, making sure to flip halfway through cooking.

Nutrition: CALORIES: 256; FAT: 9G; PROTEIN: 39G; SUGAR: 5G

Potato Crusted Salmon

Preparation Time: 10 minutes

Cooking Time: 15 minutes

Serving: 4

Ingredients

- 1pound salmon, swordfish, or arctic char fillets, 3/4 inch thick

- egg white

- 2tablespoons water

- 1/3 cup dry instant mashed potatoes

- 2teaspoons cornstarch

- 1teaspoon paprika

- 1teaspoon lemon pepper seasoning

Directions:

1. Remove and skin from the fish and cut it into four serving pieces. Mix the egg white and water. Mix all of the dry ingredients. Dip the fillets into the egg white mixture, then press into the potato mix to coat evenly.

2. Pour into the Oven rack/basket. Place the Rack on the middle-shelf of the Smart Air Fryer Oven. Set temperature to 360°F, and set time to 15 minutes, flip the filets halfway through.

Nutrition: CALORIES: 176; FAT: 7G; PROTEIN: 23G; 5G

Salmon Croquettes

Preparation Time: 10 minutes

Cooking Time: 10 minutes

Serving: 7

Ingredients

- Panko breadcrumbs
- Almond flour
- 2egg whites
- 2tbsp. chopped chives
- 2 tbsp. minced garlic cloves
- ½ C. chopped onion
- 2/3 C. grated carrots
- 1pound chopped salmon fillet

Directions:

1. Mix all ingredients minus breadcrumbs, flour, and egg whites.

1. Shape mixture into balls. Then coat them in flour, then egg, and then breadcrumbs. Drizzle with olive oil.

2. Pour the coated salmon balls into the Oven rack/basket. Place the Rack on the middle-shelf of the Smart Air Fryer Oven. Set temperature to 350°F, and set time to 6 minutes. Shake and cook an additional 4 minutes until golden in color.

Nutrition: CALORIES: 503; CARBS: 61g; FAT: 9G; PROTEIN: 5G; SUGAR: 4G

Snapper Scampi

Preparation Time: 5 minutes

Cooking Time: 10 minutes

Serving: 4

Ingredients

- 4(6-ounce) skinless snapper or arctic char fillets
- 1tablespoon olive oil
- 3tablespoons lemon juice, divided
- ½ teaspoon dried basil
- Pinch salt
- Freshly ground black pepper
- tablespoons butter
- cloves garlic, minced

Directions:

1. Rub the fish fillets with olive oil and one tablespoon of lemon juice. Sprinkle with the basil, salt, pepper, and place in the Smart Air Fryer Oven basket.

2. Grill the fish for 7 to 8 minutes or until the fish just flakes when tested with a fork. Remove the fish from the basket and put on a serving plate. Cover to keep warm. In a 6-by-6-by-2-inch pan, combine the butter, remaining two tablespoons lemon juice, and garlic. Cook in the Smart Air Fryer Oven for 1 to 2 minutes or until the garlic is sizzling. Pour this mixture over the fish and serve.

Nutrition: CALORIES: 265; CARBS: 1g; FAT: 11G; PROTEIN: 39G; FIBER: 0G

The Fish Cakes With Mango Relish

Preparation Time: 5 minutes

Cooking Time: 10 minutes

Serving: 4

Ingredients

- 1 lb. White Fish Fillets

- 3 Tbsps. Ground Coconut

- 1 Ripened Mango

- ½ Tips. Chili Paste

- 1Tbsps Fresh Parsley

- 1Green Onion

- 1 Lime

- 1 Tsp. Salt

- 1 Egg

Directions:

1   To make the relish, peel and dice the mango into cubes. Combine with a half teaspoon of chili paste, a tablespoon of parsley, and

the zest and juice of half a lime.

1   In a food processor, pulse the fish
until it forms a smooth texture. Place into a bowl
and add the salt, egg, chopped green onion,
parsley, two tablespoons of the coconut, and the
remainder of the chili paste and lime zest and juice.
Combine well

2   Portion the mixture into ten
equal balls and flatten them into small patties. Pour
the reserved tablespoon of the coconut onto a dish
and roll the cakes over to coat.

3   Preheat the Smart Air Fryer
Oven to 390 degrees

2   Place the fish cakes into the
Smart Air Fryer Oven and cook for 8 minutes. They
should be crisp and lightly browned when ready

4   Serve hot with mango
relish

Air Fryer Fish Tacos

Preparation Time: 5 minutes

Cooking Time: 15 minutes

Serving: 4

Ingredients

- 1 pound cod
- 1 tbsp. cumin
- ½ tbsp. chili powder
- 1 ½ C. almond flour
- 1 ½ C. coconut flour
- 10 ounces Mexican beer
- 2eggs

Directions:

1. Whisk beer and eggs together.

2. Whisk flours, pepper, salt, cumin, and chili powder together.

3. Slice cod into large pieces and coat in egg mixture then flour mixture.

4. Spray bottom of your Smart Air Fryer Oven basket with olive oil and add coated

codpieces. Cook 15 minutes at 375 degrees.

5. Serve on lettuce leaves topped with homemade salsa.

Nutrition: CALORIES: 178; CARBS: 61g; FAT: 10G; PROTEIN: 19G; SUGAR: 1G

Firecracker Shrimp

Preparation Time: 10 minutes

Cooking Time: 8 minutes

Serving: 4

Ingredients

For the shrimp

- 1 pound raw shrimp, peeled and deveined

- Salt

- Pepper

- One egg

- ½ cup all-purpose flour

- ¾ cup panko bread crumbs

- Cooking oil

For the firecracker sauce

- ⅓   cup sour cream

- 2tablespoons Sriracha

- ¼ cup sweet chili sauce

Directions:

1. Season the shrimp with salt and pepper to taste. In a small cup, beat the egg.

2. In another small bowl, place the flour. In a third small bowl, add the panko bread crumbs.

3. Spray the Smart Air Fryer Oven basket with cooking oil.

4. Dip the shrimp in the flour, then the egg, and then the bread crumbs. Place the shrimp in the air fryer basket. It is okay to stack them. Spray the shrimp with cooking oil.

5. Cook for 4 minutes. Open the Smart Air Fryer Oven and flip the shrimp. I recommend scanning individually instead of shaking to keep the breading intact— Cook for an additional 4 minutes or until crisp.

6. While the shrimp is cooking, make the firecracker sauce: In a small bowl, combine the sour cream, Sriracha, and sweet chili sauce. Mix well. Serve with the shrimp.

Nutrition:

CALORIES: 266; CARBS: 23g; FAT: 6G; PROTEIN: 27G; FIBER: 1G

Sesame Seeds Coated Fish

Preparation Time: 10 minutes

Cooking Time: 8minutes

Serving: 5

Ingredients

- 3tablespoons plain flour

- 2eggs

- ½ cup sesame seeds, toasted

- ½ cup breadcrumbs

- 1/8 teaspoon dried rosemary, crushed

- Pinch of salt

- Pinch of black pepper

- 3tablespoons olive oil

- 5frozen fish fillets (white fish of your choice)

Directions:

1. Place the flour in a shallow dish. In a second shallow dish, beat the eggs. In a third shallow dish, add remaining ingredients except for fish fillets and mix till a crumbly mixture forms.

2. Coat the fillets with flour and shake off the excess flour.

3. Then, dip the fillets in an egg.

4. Then coat the fillets with sesame seeds mixture generously.

5. Preheat the Smart Air Fryer Oven to 390 degrees F.

6. Line an Air fryer basket with a piece of foil. Arrange the fillets into a prepared basket.

7. Cook for about 14 minutes, flipping once after 10 minutes.

Bacon-Wrapped Scallops

Preparation Time: 5 minutes

Cooking Time: 5minutes

Serving: 4

Ingredients

- 5slices of center-cut bacon

- 20 raw sea scallops   1 tsp. paprika

- 1tsp. lemon pepper

Directions:

1. Rinse and drain scallops, placing on paper towels to soak up excess moisture.

1. Cut slices of bacon into four pieces.

2. Wrap each scallop with a piece of bacon, using toothpicks to secure. Sprinkle wrapped scallops with paprika and lemon pepper.

3. Spray air fryer basket with olive oil and add scallops.

4. Cook 5-6 minutes at 400 degrees, making sure to flip halfway through.

Nutrition:

CALORIES: 389; CARBS: 63g; FAT: 17G; PROTEIN: 21G; SUGAR: 1G

Korean Chicken Wings

Preparation Time: 5 minutes

Cooking Time: 10 minutes

Serving: 8

Ingredients

Wings:

- 1 tsp. pepper

- 1 tsp. salt

- 2 pounds of chicken wings

Sauce:

- Two packets Splenda

- 1 tbsp. minced garlic

- 1 tbsp. minced ginger

- 1 tbsp. sesame oil

- 1 tsp. agave nectar

- 1 tbsp. mayo

- 2 tbsp. gochujang

Finishing:

- ¼ C. chopped green onions

- 2 tsp. sesame seeds

Directions:

1. Ensure air fryer oven is preheated to 400 degrees.

2. Line a small pan with foil, place a rack onto the pan, and then put it into the air fryer oven.

3. Season wings with pepper and salt and place onto the rack.

4. Set temperature to 160°F, set time to 20 minutes, and air fry 20 minutes, turning at 10 minutes.

5. As chicken air fries, mix all the sauce components.

6. Once a thermometer says that the chicken has reached 160 degrees, take out wings and a bowl.

7. Pour half of the sauce mixture over wings, tossing well to coat.

8. Put coated wings back into air fryer for 5 minutes or till they reach 165 degrees.

9. Remove and sprinkle with green onions and sesame seeds. Dip into an extra sauce.

NUTRITION:

CALORIES: 356

FAT: 26G

PROTEIN:23G

SUGAR:2G

Almond Flour Coco-Milk Battered Chicken

Preparation Time: 5 minutes

Cooking Time: 30 minutes

Serving: 4

Ingredients

- ¼ cup of coconut milk

- ½ cup almond flour

- 1 ½ tablespoon old bay Cajun seasoning

- One egg, beaten

- Four small chicken thighs

- Salt and pepper to taste

Directions:

1. Preheat the air fryer oven for 5 minutes.

2. Mix the egg and coconut milk in a bowl.

3. Soak the chicken thighs in the beaten egg mixture.

4. In a mixing bowl, combine the almond flour, Cajun seasoning, salt, and pepper.

5. Dredge the chicken thighs in the almond flour mixture.

6. Place in the air fryer basket.

7. Cook for 30 minutes at 350°F.

NUTRITION:

CALORIES: 590; FAT: 38G; PROTEIN: 32.5G; CARBS: 3.2G

Sweet And Sour Chicken

Preparation Time: 20 minutes

Cooking Time: 25 minutes

Serving: 6

Ingredients

- 3 Chicken Breasts, cubed
- 1/2 Cup Flour
- 1/2 Cup Cornstarch
- 2 Red Peppers, sliced
- 1Onion, chopped
- 2 Carrots, julienned
- 3/4 Cup Sugar
- 2 Tbsps. Cornstarch
- 1/3 Cup Vinegar
- 2/3 Cup Water
- 1/4 cup Soy sauce
- 1 Tbsp. Ketchup

Directions:

1. Preheat the air fryer oven to 375 degrees.

2. Combine the flour, cornstarch, and chicken in an airtight container and shake to combine

3. Remove chicken from the container and shake off any excess flour.

4. Add chicken to the Air Fryer tray and cook for 20 minutes.

5. In a saucepan, whisk together sugar, water, vinegar, soy sauce, and ketchup. Bring to a boil over medium heat, reduce the heat, then simmer for 2 minutes

6. After cooking the chicken for 20 minutes, add the vegetables and sauce mixture to the air fryer oven and cook for another 5 minutes

7. Serve over hot rice

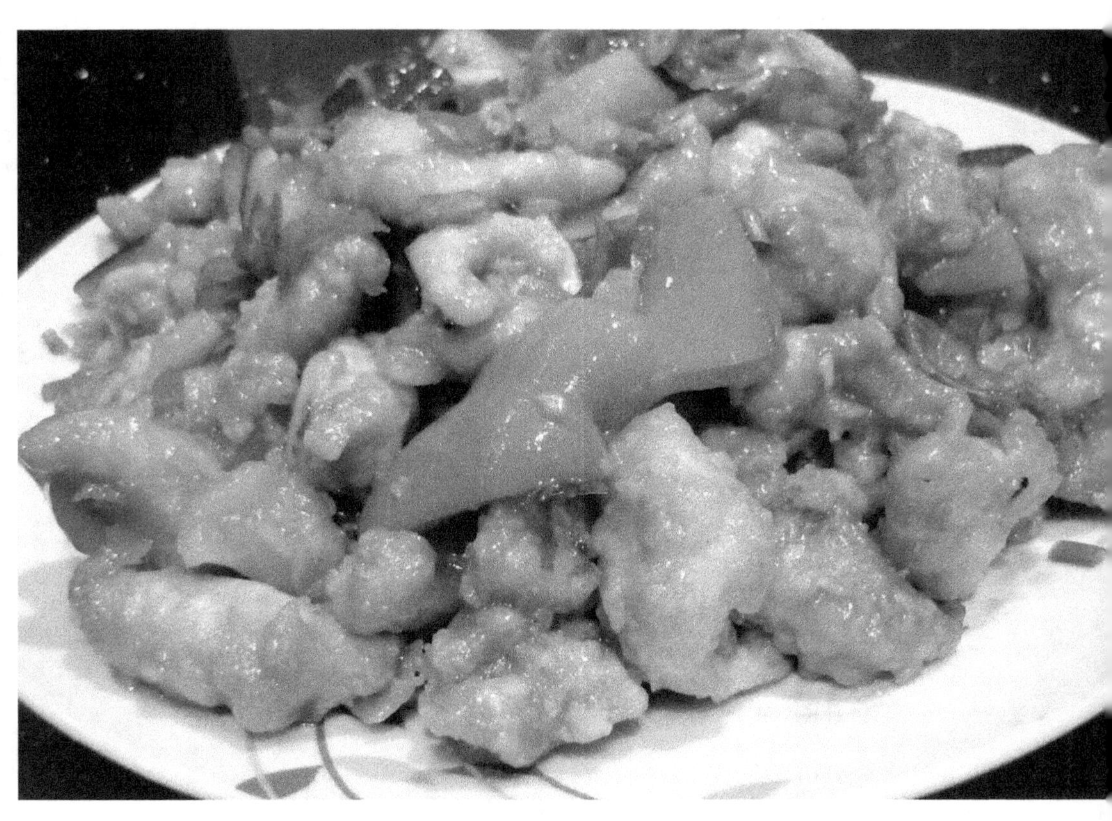